I0442127

Multiple Sclerosis

Diet for Recovery

The Multiple Sclerosis Autoimmune Disease Recovery Diet Guide for Beginners

All Rights Reserved. No part of this publication may be reproduced in any form or by any means, including scanning, photocopying, or otherwise without prior written permission of the copyright holder. Copyright © 2014

Table of Contents

Introduction

Multiple Sclerosis is a lifelong challenging disease. You sometimes lose the feeling in your legs, or lose body coordination, sometimes you have hazy or double vision, and sometimes you just collapse to the floor. You don't really feel anything at all even at the point when you're already going down. It's like the world suddenly stops right then and there. It's like you just begin to feel like floating and there's nothing there beneath you.

Those are just some of the things that people with **Multiple Sclerosis** (or MS) have to live with their entire lives. But even if some of their life functions have been limited, people with MS still see life as a gift that should be appreciated. They learn to appreciate what most people ignore.

Understanding MS – Its Nature and Symptoms

Multiple Sclerosis is a condition that is known by various names. Some people call it encephalomyelitis disseminate while others refer to it as disseminated sclerosis. Experts have classified it as a type of inflammatory disease. It basically affects certain parts of a patient's nervous system.

Both the brain and the spinal cord are damaged by this disease, specifically the insulating covers of the nerve cells in both organs. This process is called demyelination since it is the myelin of the nerves that is being destroyed.

The nervous system is basically made out of nerves. Simply put, the entire nervous system acts as a message relay system for the entire human body. The nerves are covered by myelin, a fatty substance that not only acts as a kind of insulation but it also helps the nerves in transmitting signals from the brain to different parts of the body. When that gets damaged, a lot of things in the body start to malfunction.

Given the scope of the damage that this disease makes, the signs and symptoms are also quite diverse. Some symptoms are psychiatric in nature while others are physical. In some patients, they get both types of symptoms.

The name of this disease (i.e. sclerosis) basically describes the scar tissue buildup that form in the brain or the spine. Sometimes the buildup is found in both of these organs. This scar tissue is also referred to as plaques.

Some of the symptoms that patients experience are progressive in nature. This means that the symptoms that patients experience build or progress over time. On the other hand, there are also symptoms that are isolated in nature, which take the form of a relapse. In such cases, the symptoms do not develop in time.

People should understand that the symptoms of this disease tend to vary from one patient to the other. Sometimes the symptoms that a single patient experiences also change as time goes by. However, there are common symptoms during the early stages which can be identified such as eye pain, double vision, weakness in the muscles, and reduced movement coordination. Some of the more advanced symptoms that have been reported include difficulty controlling one's urination, spasticity, and certain cognition difficulties.

Causes of **Multiple Sclerosis**

Medical experts often label MS as a mysterious disease. Some even call it a frustrating disease. It is actually one of the diseases that have unknown causes. What is known so far is that patient's immune system has failed and that the very immune system of a patient is attacking and damaging healthy nerves. Because of this, MS is classified as an autoimmune disease. However, the cause of this failure still needs to be identified.

Take note that the brain or the nerves of the brain and spine has the ability to replenish its myelin. However, in the case of MS, the nerves aren't able to keep up with the deterioration that is occurring. That is part and parcel of this condition.

Patients Turning to Dietary Solutions

It is an interesting trend that MS patients are turning to diets and other alternative treatments. Medical experts nowadays have observed that there are patients who experienced improvements in their conditions after making certain dietary changes.

It is rather unfortunate that a lot of marketing gimmicks have popped up declaring that certain foods can actually cure MS. Others are a bit more conservative saying that this or that diet can help treat the disease. Whenever you read a statement making that sort of claim, remember that the medical world still has to decide on the matter.

Nevertheless, there are those like Dr. Ellen Mowry from Johns Hopkins University who observed that diet does have an impact on the many different symptoms associated with MS as well as other autoimmune diseases. Some even believe that dietary changes can help in the treatment of **Multiple Sclerosis**.

As a bit of a caveat to this discussion, you should remember that studies about the effects of diet on MS patients are still ongoing. Furthermore, there is still a lot of research that still needs to be done. That is why people like Heidi Crayton, MD (MS Center of Greater Washington) has stated that not one medical expert knows for sure which diet will absolutely work for all patients.

Some diets work for some patients but it is not a guarantee that it will work for you. There are patients who undergo a certain diet and the symptoms are slowly alleviated. In time the quality of their lives has been improved. However, there are also those who try the very same diet but it does completely nothing for them.

This is one of the reasons why some people get frustrated over this disease. Thus the National Multiple Sclerosis Society has issued a warning for all patients that they shouldn't believe every diet that is touted as a cure all for this disease. Since the studies are still inconclusive, people should bear in mind that there is still no diet that can cure this disease or get rid of all symptoms.

What medical practitioners are saying is that certain dietary changes have been observed as being beneficial for patients. The reason behind why they work is as much a mystery as the disease itself. A handful of studies are showing some promise but nothing is yet that solid or absolutely conclusive.

For instance, a low saturated fat diet plus omega 3 fatty acid supplements showed pretty good results. However, when the said study was reviewed, the results weren't confirmed in the review. This is the reason the results for that study are rather inconclusive for now. That is where it stands until further studies can be performed.

Some experts have also theorized and observed that Vitamin D supplements may help alleviate or treat the symptoms associated with this disease. Statistics show that there are more MS patients who live in areas of the world that have lesser exposure to sunlight; thus the theory that they might be lacking Vitamin D.

They tried it with some patients and it seemed to work to a certain degree where doctors have begun to believe that there is strong evidence in support of this treatment approach. However, the very same doctors who performed the said treatment still shrug their shoulders and admit that they still need to make this study conclusive. Their advice is that patients should still see their doctor, determine their current blood Vitamin D levels, and ask their doctors how much Vitamin D supplements they should take.

Certain Dietary Changes that May Help MS Patients

- Avoid any kind of extreme diet especially the ones that haven't been tested. Remember that a diet can and will change the way a person eat. Given the current well-being of MS patients, a drastic dietary change can be harmful to them. Medical experts consider going on a diet as something similar to actually taking medication. Treat untested diet like an untested drug, which is why experts always tell people to check with their doctors.

- Eating balanced and nutritious meals is absolutely beneficial to patients according to representatives of the **Multiple Sclerosis Society UK**. Meals that provide balanced nutrition helps the body work at its fullest. This is absolutely beneficial for those who have to bear with long term conditions and unpredictable symptoms. Some patients may want to take supplements but they recommend that getting your vitamins and minerals through the food you eat is still the best way for patients.

  A balanced diet helps patients control their weight, reduce the risk of complications, increases flexibility, decreases fatigue, strengthens the heart, reduces the risk of developing skin problems, avoid skin problems, helps keeps your teeth and gums healthy, and helps maintain normal bladder function and bowel movement.

- Reduce fat intake and increase the amount of fiber in your diet. Cutting back on fat benefits everyone and not just MS patients. Most people's diets nowadays are loaded with saturated fats and are low in fiber. Increasing the fiber content in the food you eat also improves overall health and prevents heart disease.

Analyzing Some of the Diets Promoted as Treatment for MS

There are many diets that have been suggested or marketed as a treatment for **Multiple Sclerosis**. Some of them have actually been tested while others still need to be verified. What follows after are some of the diets that have been used and tried by MS patients.

Each of these diets has their benefits and shortcomings as well. It should be noted that none of these diets are 100% recommended by the entire medical community. Some MS organizations may have tried or studied one or two of these diets but it is not an assurance that the results are nothing short of conclusive.

The Swank Diet

If you're looking for the most popular diet that deals with **Multiple Sclerosis** then the Swank Diet is definitely that diet. This diet was developed for quite a while now. It was introduced by Dr. Roy Swank back in the 1940's. This diet is based on his studies in low saturated fat.

Dr. Swank's study involved 150 patients and all of them had to take low saturated fat diets. One of the downsides of this study is that there is no control group to compare with. This means there wasn't another group of patients who did not have low saturated fat diets.

Dr. Swank actually kept meticulous records and he tested his patients regularly. Partly good news, many of the patients were not able to stick to this diet. The records were continued until about 34 years into the lives of these patients, which is quite extensive. The data also include relapse records, which is interesting.

The study was supported by grants Canada's MS Society, Canada's Department of Health, and other grants from other institutions as well. Several medical papers came out of this research. The said papers were published in several medical journals including the Lancet.

Dr. Swank reports that the patients who participated in the diet only consumed 16 grams of saturated fat each day. That is an average amount per day. On the other hand, he also reports that the patients who were not able to adhere to the diet had 38 grams of saturated fat each day.

Take note that 38 grams of saturated fat is already a big improvement in the lives of those patients. The average human consumption of saturated fat nowadays is 125 grams per day on average. However, he also admits that the best results were obtained from those who had very minimal disability. Throughout this study 58 of the 72 who were not able to stick to their diets were already dead after 34 years. 45 out of the 58 participants died due to MS related causes.

95 percent of the participants in this study survived after 34 years have passed. More good news is that all of the patients who survived were able to continue active lives. The statistics for this group excludes those who have died from non-MS causes years later. Now, even with such promising results this study still needs to be verified.

Even though the study seems promising the diet still has to show some convincing benefits. After being reviewed by peers, the results still aren't conclusive. Another drawback of this diet is the fact that it is really hard to stick to and patients will probably back away from the diet eventually.

Gluten Free Diet

Another popular diet that has been promoted as a possible treatment for **Multiple Sclerosis** is the gluten free diet. This diet may have become popular but the tests show no beneficial results. A review was conducted by representatives from the Colorado Neurological Institute and the reviewers were not convinced. They were not able to verify the claims of this diet.

Wahls Diet

Some people may call Wahls Diet as vegetarian diet due to the fact that it emphasizes heavily on the consumption of fruits and vegetables. You can compare the Wahls Diet to the diet segment of the OMS Program. They have a few similarities except that the Wahls Diet does not recommend the use of supplements.

The main bulk of a patient's diet in Wahls is nine cups of fruits and veggies. Experts and reviewers of this diet say there is nothing potentially wrong with eating that amount of vegetables and fruits. In fact it can very well be beneficial to MS patients all in all. And just like the other diets reviewed here, the Wahls Diet still has to provide convincing and otherwise conclusive results before any recommendations can be made in its favor.

Best Bet Diet

The Best Bet Diet is one of the popular diets advertised for **Multiple Sclerosis** today. It's one that you will hardly miss if you look for diets that are suitable for MS patients. Medical experts and MS societies and organizations may not have confirmed the efficacy of this diet but the components of this diet are pretty much what they recommend to most patients.

This diet actually recommends different kinds of food sources, which includes red meat, dairy, and grains. The diet puts a high premium on low fat meat sources including fish, chicken, and turkey (mostly white meat sources but there are red meat sources as well).

The diet also includes a recommendation for allergy testing just to be sure that patients are not ingesting food that they are allergic to. Other than the recommended food, the diet also includes 18 different supplements that patients are supposed to consume.

This diet still has to show some conclusive results during tests. Just like the Swank Diet, this diet provides patients with very low energy. Patients who are already underweight may have difficulty staying within this diet's regimen.

Why Do These Diets Work

The main reason why these diets have very positive results remains unknown. One common denominator of these diets is the fact that they recommend very low saturated fat intake. That pretty much benefits everyone whether they have **Multiple Sclerosis** or not.

However, the reduced fat intake has an added benefit for MS patients. You see dietary fats have a huge role in the progression of this disease. The more fats a patient eats the worse the condition gets. That is why medical experts agree that patients should reduce their intake of dietary fats.

The bottom line from a dietary point of view here is for patients to cut down on their consumption of saturated fats. Studies about the effect of polyunsaturated fatty acids on the central nervous system are still undergoing and more time is needed to make any findings.

Some argue that the consumption of fats has a huge role in the development of neurological and autoimmune diseases. They even expect that those who are critical of this view will one day come to accept it as fact.

In the second segment of this book, you will find a collection of recipes that are designed to aid in the recovery process of **Multiple Sclerosis** as well as other autoimmune related disease.

Breakfast Ideas

Amazon Smoothie

Prep time: 5 minutes

INGREDIENTS

1 handful spinach

½ avocado

1 banana

1 large stalk celery

1 tsp cinnamon

1 cup water

INSTRUCTIONS

1. Slice avocado in half and remove the nut. Break the banana into small pieces and chop the celery into small pieces.
2. Combine all ingredients except for the spinach into a blender. Blend them until pureed, then add spinach and blend until pureed. Serve or chill and then serve.

Green Goodness Smoothie

Prep Time: 5 minutes

INGREDIENTS

2 cups spinach

2 whole kale leaves (1 cup chopped)

1 banana

1 green apple

1/2 cup green grapes

1 cup water (or fresh nut milk)

INSTRUCTIONS

1. Remove stems and ribs from kale. Core apple and dice. Peel banana.
2. Add water, banana and grapes to full sized blender. Process until solids are broken down.
3. Add greens and pulse on low for 30 seconds to break down. Then process on high for 1 minute, until smooth.
4. Pour into serving glasses and serve immediately.
5. Or chill in refrigerator for 20 minutes, blend for a few seconds to incorporate separated liquid, then pour into serving glasses and serve chilled.

Northern Typhoon

Prep time: 5 minutes

INGREDIENTS

1 handful Kale

1 banana

1 large cucumber

1 handful green beans

1 tsp cinnamon

1 cup water

INSTRUCTIONS

1. Break the banana into small pieces. De-stem the kale, skin and chop the cucumber and de-stem the green beans.
2. Combine all ingredients except for kale in a blender. Blend them until pureed, then add kale and blend until pureed. Serve or chill and then serve.

Pineapple Coconut Smoothie

Prep Time: 10 minutes*

INSTRUCTIONS

1 fresh coconut (or 1/2 cup flaked coconut)

1/2 cup pineapple chunks (fresh or frozen)

1 cup ice (crushed preferably)

Water

DIRECTIONS

1. *Soak flaked coconut in 1 1/2 cups water in refrigerator overnight, if using.
2. Add soaked coconut and soaking liquid to high-speed blender. Or remove flesh from fresh coconut and add to high-speed blender with 1 1/2 cups water. Process until well blended and fairly smooth, about 1 - 2 minutes.
3. Strain mixture through nut milk bag, cheesecloth or strainer back into blender.
4. Reserve pulp and set aside to dry and dehydrate, then use as coconut flour.
5. Cut pineapple flesh from peel, then chop. Add to blender with ice. Process until smooth, about 1 - 2 minutes.
6. Pour into serving glass and serve immediately.

Sweet Citrus Salad with Coconut Cream

Prep Time: 10 minutes

Servings: 1

INSTRUCTIONS

1 fresh coconut (or 1/2 cup flaked coconut)

1/4 - 1/3 cup dried pitted dates

1 blood orange

1 tangerine (or navel orange or clementine)

1/2 grapefruit (ruby red, pink or white)

1/2 lime

Water

INGREDIENTS

1. *Soak flaked coconut in 1 cup water overnight in refrigerator, if using. Soak dates in enough water to cover overnight in refrigerator. Drain.

2. Add soaked coconut and soaking liquid to high-speed blender. Or remove flesh from fresh coconut and add to high-speed blender with 3/4 cup water. Process until thick and fairly smooth, about 1 - 2 minutes.

3. Strain mixture through nut milk bag, cheesecloth or strainer back into blender or to food processor.

4. Reserve pulp and set aside to dry and dehydrate, then use as coconut flour.

5. Add soaked dates to processor and process until smooth. Set aside.

6. Peel all citrus and cut into segments. Add to serving dish. Top with sweet coconut cream.

7. Serve immediately. Or refrigerate 20 minutes and serve chilled.

Lunch and Dinner Ideas

Roasted Turkey Legs

Prep Time: 10 minutes*

Cook Time: 1 hour 20 minutes

Servings: 4

INGREDIENTS

2 large turkey legs

1/2 teaspoon garlic powder

1/2 teaspoon onion powder

1/2 teaspoon dried rosemary

1/2 teaspoon dried thyme

1/2 teaspoon Celtic sea salt

1 1/2 tablespoon coconut oil

Brine

4 cups water

1/4 cup Celtic sea salt

1/4 cup date butter

INSTRUCTIONS

1. *For *Brine*, add water, salt and date butter to wide, shallow container. Mix to combine. Add turkey legs and submerge completely in *Brine*. Marinate in refrigerator 12 - 24 hours.

2. Preheat oven to 350 degrees F. Place wire rack over sheet pan.

3. Remove turkey legs from brine. Rub salt, spices and oil over turkey legs, and under skin.

4. Place coated turkey legs on wire rack and bake about 35 - 40 minutes. Carefully turn turkey legs over and bake another 35 - 40 minutes, until skin is crisp and meat is cooked through.

5. Remove from oven and let rest about 2 minutes. Then serve hot.

Highland Beef Haggis

Prep Time: 10 minutes

Cook Time: 3 hours

Servings: 4

INGREDIENTS

8 oz (1/2 lb) ground beef (or bison, elk, etc.)

8 oz (1/2 lb) lamb shoulder

4 oz (1/4 lb) calves liver

2 onions (yellow or white)

1/2 head cauliflower (about 1 cup riced)

1 cup beef stock

2 garlic cloves

1/2 teaspoon ground nutmeg

1/4 teaspoon ground coriander

1/2 teaspoon Celtic sea salt

1/4 cup coconut oil

Water

INSTRUCTIONS

1. Preheat oven to 300 degrees F. Generously coat baking dish with coconut oil.
2. Add liver to small pan with enough water to cover over high heat. Bring to simmer and cook about 5 minutes. Drain and set aside to cool.

3. Roughly chop cauliflower. Peel and roughly chop onions and garlic. Add to food processor with lamb shoulder and par-cooked liver. Process until coarsely ground, about 2 minutes.

4. Add ground beef, stock, salt, and spices and pulse to combine. Transfer to prepared baking dish and cover tightly with aluminum foil.

5. Place covered dish in roasting pan. Add water to roasting pan 3/4 of the way up side of baking dish.

6. Bake for 3 hours. Remove from oven and carefully remove foil. Let rest about 10 minutes.

7. Remove baking dish from roasting pan. To plate, place serving dish over baking dish and carefully invert. Slice haggis into wedges and serve hot.

Bacon Wrapped Filet Mignon

Prep Time: 5 minutes

Cook Time: 20 minutes

Servings: 2

INGREDIENTS

2 (6 oz each) filet mignon steaks

2 thick slices nitrate-free bacon

Celtic sea salt, to taste

1 tablespoon coconut oil (optional)

Toothpicks

INSTRUCTIONS

1. Preheat oven to 350 degrees F. Heat medium oven-safe pan or skillet over medium heat.

2. Add bacon to hot pan. Cook and render out fat for about 5 minutes, until about halfway cooked. Remove bacon from pan and set aside, reserving bacon fat in pan. Add coconut oil to pan, if desired.

3. Wrap par-cooked bacon around steaks and secure with toothpick. Sprinkle steaks with salt to taste.

4. Add wrapped seasoned steaks to hot oiled pan and sear 2 minutes per side. Carefully flip half way through cooking.

5. Remove pan from stove and place in preheated oven. Cook about 8 - 10 minutes, until bacon is cooked through and steak is medium-rare.

6. Remove steaks from oven and transfer to cutting board. Set aside and let rest at least 2 minutes.

7. Transfer to serving dish and serve hot.

Herb Roasted Pork Tenderloin

Prep Time: 10 minutes*

Cook Time: 15 minutes

Servings: 4

INGREDIENTS

1 pork tenderloin

1 teaspoon dried rosemary

1 teaspoon dried thyme

1 teaspoon dried oregano

1 teaspoon dried basil

1 teaspoon dried marjoram (optional)

1 teaspoon Celtic sea salt

Apricot Sauce

1 cup dried apricots

2/3 cup water

1 teaspoon apple cider vinegar (or dry white wine)

INSTRUCTIONS

1. Preheat oven to 425 degrees F. Heat small pan over medium heat.

2. Rub tenderloin with salt and spices, then press into meat so it adheres. Place on sheet pan, or wire rack over sheet pan.

3. Roast for 10 - 15 minutes, until just cooked through and no pink remains. Remove pork from oven and let rest 10 minutes.

4. For *Apricot Sauce*, add dried apricots, water and vinegar to food processor or high-speed blender. Process until smooth, about 1 - 2 minutes.

5. Add *Apricot Sauce* to hot pan and reduce until slightly thickened. Stir well and do not let burn. Remove from heat.

6. Slice pork and transfer to serving dish. Top pork with *Apricot Sauce* and serve warm.

Classic Churrasco with Chimichurri

Prep Time: 10 minutes*

Cook Time: 5 minutes

Servings: 4

INGREDIENTS

24 oz (1 1/2 lb) beef tenderloin

Chimichurri

1 cup coconut oil

1/3 cup apple cider vinegar (or coconut aminos)

1/3 cup water

1 large bunch cilantro

1 large bunch parsley

1/2 cup fresh mint leaves

6 garlic cloves

1 teaspoon Celtic sea salt

INSTRUCTIONS

1. For *Chimichurri*, peel garlic and add to food processor or high-speed blender. Remove cilantro, parsley and mint leaves from stems. Add to processor and process to finely chop, about 1 minute. Add oil, water, salt and spices. Process until thick sauce forms, about 1 - 2 minutes.

2. Cut tenderloin lengthwise into 4 even slices, then flatten with tenderizing or kitchen mallet to 1/2 inch thickness. Place meat in between two parchment sheets to flatten, if preferred.

3. *Pour 1/4 of the *Chimichurri* into a baking dish just large enough to fit tenderloin. Place beef over *Chimichurri*, then top with second 1/4 of *Chimichurri*. Set aside to marinate about 1 hour. Transfer remaining *Chimichurri* to serving dish.

4. Heat grill or grated skillet over high heat.

Moist Roasted Turkey

Prep Time: 10 minutes*

Cook Time: 4 - 6 hours

Servings: 12

INGREDIENTS

20 lb (approx.) whole turkey

2 teaspoons Celtic sea salt

2 tablespoons coconut oil

Brine

1 - 2 gallons water

1 cup Celtic sea salt

1 cup date butter

INSTRUCTIONS

1. *For *Brine*, add 1/2 gallon of water, salt and date butter to large baking dish or roasting pan. Mix to combine. Remove any entrails from turkey and add to *Brine*, plus and enough water to submerge completely. Marinate in refrigerator 12 - 24 hours.

2. Preheat oven to 350 degrees F. Place roasting rack in clean roasting pan.

3. Drain turkey and rub salt and oil over and under skin, where possible.

4. Place seasoned turkey on roasting rack and bake about 15 - 18 minutes per lb, about 5 hours for 20 lb bird. Or until internal

temperature reaches 165 degrees F. Baste with rendered fat and juices throughout cooking for even browning.

5. Remove turkey from oven and let rest 20 - 30 minutes.
6. Carve and serve warm.

Quick Raw Avocado Slaw

Prep Time: 10 minutes*

Cook Time: 20 minutes

Servings: 4

INGREDIENTS

1/2 head cabbage (2 cups shredded)

1 avocado

1 carrot

Zest of 1 lemon

Juice of 1 lemon

1 tablespoon raw honey

2 tablespoons apple cider vinegar

1 teaspoon sea salt

INSTRUCTIONS

1. Cut avocado in half and remove pit. Scoop flesh into large mixing bowl and mash with fork.

2. Remove any tough outer leaves and core from cabbage. Shred cabbage and carrot. Add to bowl with vinegar, honey and salt. Zest *then* juice lemon, and add.

3. Toss to combine.

4. Serve immediately. Or and place in refrigerator for 20 minutes and serve chilled.

Snack Ideas

Smoked Salmon and Avocado Snack

Prep Time: 5* minutes

Servings: 2

INGREDIENTS

4 oz (1 or 1/2 package) cold-smoked salmon

1 avocado

1 stalk fresh dill

Pinch sea salt

1/2 lemon (optional)

INSTRUCTIONS

1. Slice avocado in half and remove pit. Cut into thick slices in peel then scoop out with large spoon.
2. Slice smoked salmon into long 1 inch strips. Wrap 1 salmon strips around each avocado slice. Arrange wrapped avocado on serving dish.
3. Mince fresh dill. Sprinkle dill and salt over avocado wraps and serve immediately.
4. Or squeeze juice of 1/2 lemon over avocado wraps, sprinkle on dill and salt, and refrigerate 20 minutes. Then serve chilled.

Olive Tapenade

Prep Time: 15 minutes

Servings: 2

INGREDIENTS

1 1/2 cups any combination pitted olives (Kalamata, Spanish, black, pimento, etc.)

2 tablespoons capers

2 anchovy fillets

1 garlic clove

2 fresh basil leaves

1/2 lemon

2 tablespoons coconut oil

INSTRUCTIONS

1. Peel garlic and add to food processor or high-speed blender. Process until finely ground.

2. Rinse and drain olives, capers and anchovy fillets. Add to processor with basil, oil and squeeze of 1/2 lemon. Process until finely chopped or coarsely ground, about 1 - 2 minutes.

3. Transfer to serving dish and serve immediately.

Spicy Tuna Tartare

Prep Time: 15* minutes

Servings: 4

INGREDIENTS

1 lb tuna steak (sushi grade)

1 small cucumber

1 ripe avocado

1 lime

1 garlic clove

2 tablespoons raw virgin coconut oil

Small bunch fresh cilantro

1 teaspoon sea salt

INSTRUCTIONS

1. Peel, seed and dice cucumber and avocado. Finely chop cilantro. Add to medium mixing bowl.
2. Remove seeds, stem and veins from hot pepper. Peel garlic and add to food processor or bullet blender. Process until smooth paste forms. Add to bowl.
3. Dice tuna, discarding any tough white gristle. Add to bowl.
4. Squeeze on lime juice and add salt.
5. Gently toss with soft spatula or large spoon.
6. Serve immediately. Or refrigerate 20 minutes and serve chilled.

Baked Candied Yams

Prep Time: 10 minutes

Cook Time: 1 hour 30 minutes

Servings: 12

INGREDIENTS

4 large sweet potatoes (yams)

1/2 cup dried pitted dates

1/4 cup dried apricots

2 tablespoons coconut butter

1 tablespoon ground cinnamon

1/2 teaspoon ground ginger

Pinch Celtic sea salt

Topping

1/4 cup date butter

INSTRUCTIONS

1. Preheat oven to 350 degrees F.
2. Gently rinse sweet potatoes and place on sheet pan.
3. Bake about 1 hour, until tender.
4. Add dates, apricots and enough water to cover in small pot. Heat over medium heat. Let simmer until water evaporates. Remove from heat.
5. Remove yams from oven and let cool about 10 minutes.

6. For *Topping*, add date butter to small pan. Heat over medium heat and cook for about 4 - 5 minutes. Stir frequently and do not burn. Remove from heat and set aside.

7. Add softened dates and apricots to large mixing bowl. Mash with potato masher, hand mixer or whisk.

8. Cut yams open lengthwise and scoop flesh into mixing bowl. Add butter, salt and spices. Mash with potato masher, hand mixer or whisk until well combined.

9. Transfer yam mixture to serving dish and top with *Topping*. Serve warm.

Lean Mean Collard Greens

Prep Time: 15 minutes

Cook Time: 2 1/2 hours

Servings: 8

INGREDIENTS

2 heads (or 2 large bags) fresh collard greens

6 slices nitrate-free bacon (or 1 small ham hock)

8 cups chicken stock

Water

INSTRUCTIONS

1. Preheat oven to 350 degrees F. Heat large pot over medium-high heat.

2. Rinse collards well and roughly chop. Place in large colander or in clean sink to drain.

3. Add bacon or ham hock to hot pot and render down for about 5 minutes.

4. Add greens to pot in batches. If all greens to not fit, reserve. Add chicken stock.

5. Bring pot to a simmer then reduce to low heat. Add any remaining greens, plus enough water just to cover, if necessary. Stir gently.

6. Simmer until collards are tender, about 2 - 2 1/2 hours.

7. Drain greens well. Transfer to serving dish and serve warm.

5. Place beef on grill or skillet on the diagonal and cook for about 1 minute, then rotate meat to create crosshatch grill marks and cook

for another minute. Then flip and repeat. Cook for about 4 minutes total for medium rare.

6. Remove from grill, slice against the grain and transfer to serving dish. Serve immediately with *Chimichurri*.

Turkey Jerky Bacon

Prep Time: 10 minutes*

Dehydrating Time: 4 - 8 hours

Servings: 4

INGREDIENTS

4 oz organic turkey (dark meat)

2 tablespoons coconut aminos (or liquid aminos)

2 tablespoons tamari (or liquid aminos or coconut aminos)

1 tablespoon lemon juice (or raw apple cider vinegar)

1 tablespoons Celtic sea salt

1/2 teaspoon garlic powder

1/2 teaspoon onion powder

INSTRUCTIONS

1. Prepare two sheet parchment. Lay one on cutting board.

2. Cut turkey into 1/4 inch strips and lay in single layer on parchment. Pound with tenderizing side of kitchen mallet. Cover turkey with second parchment sheet, then pound with flat side of tenderizing mallet to 1/8 inch thickness.

3. *Place turkey strips in medium mixing bowl or shallow dish. Add coconut aminos, tamari, lemon juice, salt and spices. Mix well to coat. Cover and place in refrigerator for 8 hours, or overnight.

4. Remove turkey from refrigerator and lay in single layer on dehydrator trays. Place trays in dehydrator and set to 120 degrees F for 4 - 8 hours.

5. After 4 hours dehydrating time, remove trays from dehydrator and test turkey by bending. If it cracks, remove and serve immediately. Or store in airtight container.
6. If still flexible, place back in dehydrator and continue dehydrating up to 4 hours, or until desired texture is achieved.

www.ingramcontent.com/pod-product-compliance
Lightning Source LLC
Chambersburg PA
CBHW070131290526
45789CB00005B/2200